DR. BARBARA 3-DAY MUCUS DETOX FOR WOMEN

Revitalize your body: Dr. Barbara's 3-days mucus cleanse tailored for women -unlock vibrant health with natural remedies and holistic wellness methods

Carlos Luz

Table of Contents

COPYRIGHT © 2023

CHAPTER ONE

Introduction to Dr. Barbara's Approach to Women's Health and Healing

In the realm of women's health and healing, Dr. Barbara's approach stands out for its comprehensive and holistic perspective. Dr. Barbara, a renowned practitioner in the field, has developed a methodology that integrates traditional medicine with modern advancements, as well as incorporates elements of alternative healing modalities. Her approach is rooted in the belief that women's health is multi-faceted, encompassing physical, mental, emotional, and spiritual well-being. In this exposition, we'll delve into the key components of Dr. Barbara's approach, examining how each aspect contributes to the overall health and healing of women.

Understanding the Holistic Framework

Central to Dr. Barbara's approach is the understanding that women's health cannot be adequately addressed by focusing solely on physical symptoms or ailments. Instead, she adopts a holistic framework that considers the interconnectedness of various aspects of a woman's life. This holistic perspective acknowledges the influence of factors such as lifestyle, environment, relationships, and emotional state on overall health. By recognizing the interplay between these elements, Dr.

Barbara aims to promote healing at a deeper level, addressing root causes rather than merely alleviating symptoms.

Empowerment Through Education

An essential aspect of Dr. Barbara's approach is empowerment through education. She believes that informed patients are better equipped to make decisions about their health and take an active role in their healing journey. To this end, Dr. Barbara emphasizes patient education, providing women with comprehensive information about their bodies, health conditions, treatment options, and self-care practices. By empowering women with knowledge, Dr. Barbara enables them to become partners in their own healthcare, fostering a sense of agency and autonomy.

Personalized Care Plans

Recognizing that each woman is unique, Dr. Barbara tailors her approach to individual needs and circumstances. Rather than adhering to a one-size-fits-all model of healthcare, she takes the time to understand each patient's health history, concerns, preferences, and goals. Based on this personalized assessment, Dr. Barbara collaborates with her patients to develop customized care plans that address their specific needs and support their overall well-being. This personalized approach ensures that women receive the most appropriate and effective treatments for their individual situations.

Integration of Conventional and Alternative Therapies

In her practice, Dr. Barbara integrates conventional medical treatments with alternative therapies, drawing from the best of both worlds. She recognizes the value of evidence-based medicine in treating acute conditions and managing chronic diseases. At the same time, Dr. Barbara also explores complementary approaches such as acupuncture, herbal medicine, massage therapy, and mind-body techniques. By combining conventional and alternative therapies, she offers her patients a comprehensive range of options for promoting health and healing.

Focus on Preventive Care

Prevention is a cornerstone of Dr. Barbara's approach to women's health and healing. Rather than waiting for illness to manifest, she emphasizes proactive measures to maintain health and prevent disease. This proactive approach may include regular screenings, vaccinations, lifestyle modifications, dietary changes, stress management techniques, and other preventive strategies. By focusing on prevention, Dr. Barbara aims to empower women to take control of their health and reduce their risk of developing serious health problems in the future.

Emotional and Psychological Support

Dr. Barbara recognizes the profound impact that emotions and psychological factors can have on women's health. She provides compassionate support and guidance to help her patients navigate the emotional and psychological aspects of their health challenges. This may involve counseling, psychotherapy, support groups, or other therapeutic interventions aimed at addressing issues such as stress, anxiety, depression, trauma, grief, and relationship problems. By addressing emotional and psychological well-being, Dr. Barbara helps her patients cultivate resilience, coping skills, and a positive outlook on life.

Promotion of Self-Care and Self-Healing

Central to Dr. Barbara's approach is the promotion of self-care and self-healing practices. She educates her patients about the importance of self-care activities such as regular exercise, healthy eating, adequate sleep, stress management, relaxation techniques, and mindfulness practices. Dr. Barbara empowers women to listen to their bodies, honor their intuition, and take proactive steps to support their own healing process. By fostering self-awareness and self-compassion, she encourages her patients to become active participants in their own health and well-being.

Community and Support Networks

Dr. Barbara recognizes the importance of community and support networks in promoting women's health and healing. She facilitates connections among her patients, providing opportunities for them to share experiences, offer mutual support, and learn from one another. This sense of community fosters a supportive environment where women feel understood, validated, and empowered to take control of their health. Dr. Barbara may also collaborate with other healthcare providers, holistic practitioners, and community organizations to enhance the support network available to her patients.

Conclusion

In conclusion, Dr. Barbara's approach to women's health and healing offers a comprehensive and holistic framework that addresses the diverse needs of women at every stage of life. By embracing a holistic perspective, empowering patients through education, providing personalized care plans, integrating conventional and alternative therapies, focusing on prevention, offering emotional and psychological support, promoting self-care and self-healing practices, and fostering community and support networks, Dr. Barbara empowers women to achieve optimal health and well-being. Her approach reflects a deep commitment to honoring the innate wisdom of the body, mind, and spirit, and supporting women in their journey toward health, healing, and wholeness.

CHAPTER TWO

Understanding the Role of Mucus in Women's Health

Mucus often evokes images of runny noses and phlegmy coughs, but its significance in women's health extends far beyond these common associations. In fact, mucus plays a crucial role in various aspects of female reproductive health, from fertility and conception to vaginal health and immune function. In this comprehensive exploration, we'll delve into the multifaceted role of mucus in women's health, shedding light on its composition, functions, and implications for overall well-being.

Composition of Female Reproductive Mucus

The mucus found in the female reproductive tract is a specialized secretion produced by the cervix and vaginal epithelium. It is composed of water, electrolytes, proteins, glycoproteins, and mucins—large, heavily glycosylated proteins that give mucus its gel-like consistency. The composition of female reproductive mucus varies throughout the menstrual cycle under the influence of estrogen and progesterone hormones.

Fertility and Conception

One of the primary functions of cervical mucus is to facilitate fertility and conception. Around the time of ovulation, under the influence of estrogen, cervical mucus becomes more abundant, thin, clear, and stretchy—resembling raw egg whites. This fertile cervical mucus creates a hospitable environment for sperm, providing nourishment, pH buffering, and protection against acidic vaginal conditions and immune factors. Sperm can swim more easily through this optimal mucus environment, increasing the likelihood of successful fertilization.

Monitoring Fertility

The changes in cervical mucus consistency and quantity throughout the menstrual cycle serve as a natural indicator of fertility. Many women use cervical mucus observations as part of fertility awareness methods (FAM) to identify their fertile window and time intercourse accordingly to maximize the chances of conception. By tracking changes in cervical mucus, women can gain insights into their menstrual cycle and reproductive health, empowering them to make informed decisions about family planning and conception.

Vaginal Health and Lubrication

In addition to its role in fertility, mucus contributes to vaginal health and lubrication. Vaginal mucus, produced by the vaginal epithelial cells and Bartholin's glands, helps maintain vaginal moisture, pH balance, and microbial balance. It serves as a natural lubricant during sexual arousal and intercourse, reducing friction and discomfort. Adequate vaginal mucus production is essential for preventing vaginal dryness, irritation, and susceptibility to infections such as yeast infections and bacterial vaginosis.

Immune Function

Mucus also plays a crucial role in immune defense within the female reproductive tract. The mucins and other components of cervical and vaginal mucus form a protective barrier against pathogens, including bacteria, viruses, and fungi. Mucus traps and immobilizes pathogens, preventing them from reaching the upper reproductive tract and causing infections. Additionally, mucus contains antimicrobial peptides and immunoglobulins that help neutralize and eliminate pathogens, bolstering the innate immune response in the vaginal environment.

Menstrual Cycle and Hormonal Influences

The production and composition of female reproductive mucus are intricately linked to the menstrual cycle and hormonal fluctuations. Estrogen, produced by the ovaries, stimulates the production of thin, watery cervical mucus during the pre-ovulatory phase, promoting fertility. Following ovulation, progesterone, released by the corpus luteum, causes cervical mucus to become thicker and less hospitable to sperm, serving as a natural barrier to prevent conception during the non-fertile phases of the menstrual cycle.

Impact of Hormonal Contraceptives

Hormonal contraceptives, such as birth control pills, patches, injections, and hormonal intrauterine devices (IUDs), can influence cervical mucus production and consistency. Some methods of hormonal contraception may thicken cervical mucus, making it more difficult for sperm to penetrate and reach the egg, thereby contributing to contraceptive effectiveness. Understanding the effects of hormonal contraceptives on cervical mucus can help women make informed choices about contraception and family planning.

Clinical Implications and Disorders

Changes in cervical mucus production, consistency, or quality may indicate underlying hormonal imbalances, infections, or reproductive disorders. For example, alterations in cervical mucus patterns may be associated with ovulatory dysfunction, polycystic ovary syndrome (PCOS), endometriosis, or cervicitis. Abnormal vaginal discharge, characterized by changes in color, odor, or texture, may signify infections such as yeast infections, bacterial vaginosis, or sexually transmitted infections (STIs). Monitoring and addressing abnormalities in cervical mucus and vaginal discharge are important for maintaining reproductive health and preventing complications.

Conclusion

In conclusion, mucus plays a vital role in women's health, particularly in the realm of reproductive health and fertility. From facilitating conception and supporting vaginal health to defending against pathogens and reflecting hormonal influences, mucus serves as a dynamic and essential component of the female reproductive tract. Understanding the functions and implications of mucus in women's health can empower women to take proactive steps to optimize their reproductive well-being and address any concerns related to fertility, vaginal health, or hormonal balance.

CHAPTER THREE

Dr. Barbara's Principles of Herbal Healing and Detoxification

Dr. Barbara's approach to herbal healing and detoxification is rooted in the belief that nature provides a wealth of botanical remedies that can support the body's innate ability to heal and cleanse. Drawing upon her extensive knowledge of herbal medicine and holistic healing practices, Dr. Barbara has developed principles and strategies to harness the therapeutic power of herbs for promoting health and vitality. In this comprehensive exploration, we'll delve into Dr. Barbara's principles of herbal healing and detoxification, examining the key concepts and practices that underpin her approach.

1. Respect for Nature and Plants

Central to Dr. Barbara's philosophy is a deep reverence for nature and the healing properties of plants. She recognizes that herbs are gifts from the earth, imbued with potent medicinal compounds and energies that can promote healing and balance in the body. Dr. Barbara emphasizes the importance of sustainable and ethical harvesting practices, ensuring that herbal remedies are sourced responsibly to minimize environmental impact and preserve biodiversity.

2. Holistic Perspective

Dr. Barbara takes a holistic approach to herbal healing and detoxification, considering the interconnectedness of body, mind, and spirit. She views health as a state of balance and harmony within the entire being, rather than merely the absence of disease. In her practice, Dr. Barbara addresses the root causes of health imbalances, taking into account physical, emotional, mental, and spiritual factors that may contribute to illness or toxicity.

3. Individualized Treatment Plans

Recognizing that each person is unique, Dr. Barbara tailors her herbal healing and detoxification protocols to individual needs and constitution. She conducts thorough assessments of her patients' health history, symptoms, lifestyle habits, and dietary patterns to determine the most appropriate herbal remedies and detoxification strategies. By customizing treatment plans, Dr. Barbara ensures that her patients receive personalized care that addresses their specific health concerns and goals.

4. Emphasis on Cleansing and Detoxification

Detoxification is a cornerstone of Dr. Barbara's approach to herbal healing, as she believes that periodic cleansing can support the body's natural detoxification pathways and enhance overall health and vitality. She advocates for gentle yet effective detoxification protocols that promote the elimination of toxins and metabolic waste products from the body, while also nourishing and rejuvenating vital organs and systems. Dr. Barbara's detoxification programs may include herbal teas, tinctures, dietary modifications, fasting, and lifestyle practices to support detoxification pathways such as liver, kidneys, lymphatic system, and colon.

5. Herbal Formulations and Preparations

Dr. Barbara utilizes a variety of herbal formulations and preparations to deliver therapeutic benefits to her patients. She selects herbs based on their specific actions and properties, such as detoxifying, immune-stimulating, anti-inflammatory, or adaptogenic effects. Common herbal preparations used by Dr. Barbara include teas, tinctures, capsules, powders, extracts, and topical applications. She may also recommend herbal formulas that combine multiple herbs synergistically to address complex health issues or support specific body systems.

6. Education and Empowerment

Empowering her patients with knowledge and understanding is a fundamental aspect of Dr. Barbara's approach to herbal healing and detoxification. She educates her patients about the properties and actions of medicinal herbs, as well as the importance of lifestyle modifications and self-care practices for maintaining health and preventing illness. By empowering her patients to take an active role in their healing journey, Dr.

Barbara fosters a sense of ownership and accountability for their health outcomes.

7. Integration with Conventional Medicine

While Dr. Barbara is a proponent of herbal medicine and natural healing modalities, she also recognizes the value of conventional medicine in certain situations. She advocates for an integrative approach to healthcare, where herbal remedies and detoxification protocols complement conventional treatments as part of a comprehensive healing strategy. Dr. Barbara collaborates with other healthcare providers to ensure coordinated care and optimize patient outcomes, prioritizing safety, efficacy, and patient preferences.

Conclusion

In conclusion, Dr. Barbara's principles of herbal healing and detoxification provide a holistic framework for promoting health, vitality, and well-being. By respecting the wisdom of nature, taking a holistic perspective, individualizing treatment plans, emphasizing cleansing and detoxification, utilizing herbal formulations, educating and empowering patients, and integrating with conventional medicine, Dr. Barbara offers a comprehensive approach to herbal healing that honors the body's innate ability to heal and thrive. Her principles reflect a commitment to nurturing health and harmony on all levels of being, supporting patients in their journey toward optimal wellness.

CHAPTER FOUR

The Importance of Addressing Mucus Imbalances in Women's Bodies

Mucus imbalances in women's bodies can have significant implications for health and well-being, impacting various aspects of reproductive health, vaginal comfort, and immune function. Understanding the importance of addressing mucus imbalances is essential for promoting optimal health and addressing underlying issues that may contribute to discomfort, infections, or fertility challenges. In this comprehensive exploration, we'll delve into the reasons why mucus imbalances in women's bodies are significant and discuss the potential consequences of untreated imbalances.

1. Impact on Fertility and Reproductive Health

One of the primary reasons why addressing mucus imbalances in women's bodies is crucial is their impact on fertility and reproductive health. Cervical mucus plays a vital role in the reproductive process by providing an optimal environment for sperm transport, survival, and fertilization. Imbalances in cervical mucus consistency, quantity, or quality can hinder sperm mobility and viability, reducing the chances of successful conception. Addressing mucus imbalances through targeted interventions and treatments can improve fertility outcomes and enhance the likelihood of achieving pregnancy for women trying to conceive.

2. Risk of Vaginal Infections

Mucus imbalances in the vaginal environment can increase the risk of vaginal infections such as bacterial vaginosis, yeast infections (candidiasis), and sexually transmitted infections (STIs). Adequate vaginal mucus production helps maintain vaginal moisture, pH balance, and microbial equilibrium, creating a protective barrier against pathogens. When mucus production is disrupted or imbalanced, the vaginal environment may become susceptible to overgrowth of harmful bacteria, fungi, or viruses, leading to infections and associated symptoms such as itching, burning, discharge, and discomfort. Addressing mucus imbalances can help restore vaginal health and reduce the risk of recurrent infections.

3. Comfort and Lubrication During Intercourse

Healthy vaginal mucus production contributes to comfort and lubrication during sexual intercourse, enhancing pleasure and reducing friction and discomfort. Insufficient mucus production or imbalances in vaginal mucus composition may result in vaginal dryness, irritation, or pain during sex, negatively impacting sexual intimacy and satisfaction. Addressing mucus imbalances can improve vaginal lubrication and comfort, enhancing sexual well-being and quality of life for women and their partners.

4. Immune Function and Protection

Mucus serves as a crucial component of the body's immune defense system, providing a physical barrier against pathogens and foreign invaders in the reproductive and respiratory tracts. Mucus contains antimicrobial peptides, immunoglobulins, and other immune factors that help neutralize and eliminate pathogens, preventing infections and supporting immune function. Imbalances in mucus production or composition can compromise the integrity of this protective barrier, making the body more susceptible to infections and inflammatory conditions. Addressing mucus imbalances can strengthen immune defenses and reduce the risk of illness and complications.

5. Overall Health and Well-Being

Maintaining balanced mucus production and composition is essential for overall health and well-being, as mucus serves various physiological functions throughout the body. In addition to its roles in fertility, vaginal health, and immune function, mucus also helps moisturize and protect mucous membranes, facilitate digestion, regulate respiratory function, and support the elimination of toxins and waste products. Addressing mucus imbalances can promote systemic health and vitality, contributing to a greater sense of well-being and vitality.

Conclusion

In conclusion, addressing mucus imbalances in women's bodies is crucial for promoting optimal health, fertility, and well-being.

Imbalances in cervical mucus, vaginal mucus, or respiratory mucus can have significant implications for fertility, reproductive health, susceptibility to infections, sexual comfort, immune function, and overall physiological balance. By recognizing the importance of mucus balance and addressing imbalances through targeted interventions, treatments, and preventive measures, women can optimize their health and reduce the risk of complications associated with mucus-related issues.

CHAPTER FIVE

Preparing Your Body and Mind for the 3-Day Herbal Mucus Cleanse

Embarking on a 3-day herbal mucus cleanse requires careful preparation of both the body and mind to ensure optimal results and a smooth detoxification process. Cleansing the body of excess mucus can promote respiratory health, alleviate congestion, enhance immune function, and support overall well-being. In this comprehensive guide, we'll explore the essential steps to prepare your body and mind for a successful herbal mucus cleanse.

1. Consultation with a Healthcare Provider

Before starting any detoxification program, it's essential to consult with a qualified healthcare provider, especially if you have any underlying health conditions or concerns. Your healthcare provider can assess your medical history, current health status, and suitability for a mucus cleanse. They can also provide personalized recommendations and guidance based on your individual needs and health goals.

2. Set Clear Intentions and Goals

Preparing your mind for a herbal mucus cleanse involves setting clear intentions and goals for the process. Take some time to reflect on why you're undertaking the cleanse and what you hope to achieve. Whether it's to improve respiratory health, boost immunity, increase energy levels, or promote overall well-being, having a clear vision of your goals can help motivate and focus your efforts throughout the cleanse.

3. Educate Yourself About Herbal Remedies

Familiarize yourself with the herbal remedies and preparations that will be used during the cleanse. Research the properties, actions, and potential benefits of the herbs included in the cleanse, as well as any possible side effects or contraindications. Understanding how each herb works and its role in the detoxification process can deepen your appreciation for the cleanse and empower you to make informed choices about your health.

4. Transition to a Clean, Whole Foods Diet

In the days leading up to the cleanse, transition to a clean, whole foods diet rich in fruits, vegetables, whole grains, legumes, nuts, seeds, and lean proteins. Minimize or eliminate processed foods, refined sugars, artificial additives, caffeine, alcohol, and other inflammatory substances that can contribute to mucus production and overall toxicity in the body. Eating a nourishing, plant-based diet will help prepare your body for the cleanse and optimize its detoxification capacity.

5. Stay Hydrated

Proper hydration is essential for supporting the body's natural detoxification processes and promoting the elimination of mucus and toxins. Drink plenty of water throughout the day to stay hydrated and facilitate mucus clearance from the respiratory tract and other tissues. You can also incorporate herbal teas, such as peppermint, ginger, or licorice root tea, which have decongestant and expectorant properties, into your daily routine to support respiratory health.

6. Practice Mindfulness and Stress Management

Preparing your mind for a herbal mucus cleanse involves practicing mindfulness and stress management techniques to promote relaxation and mental clarity. Engage in activities such as meditation, deep breathing exercises, yoga, tai chi, or nature walks to reduce stress levels, calm the mind, and cultivate a sense of inner peace. Stress can impair detoxification pathways and exacerbate mucus production, so prioritizing stress management is essential for optimizing the cleanse.

7. Gather Supplies and Create a Supportive Environment

Gather all the supplies you'll need for the cleanse, including herbal teas, tinctures, supplements, and any other detoxification aids recommended by your healthcare provider or herbalist. Create a supportive environment in your home that fosters relaxation, tranquility, and healing during the cleanse. Clear clutter, create a cozy space for rest and reflection, and surround yourself with positive affirmations and inspirational materials to uplift your spirits throughout the process.

8. Mentally Prepare for Challenges and Detox Symptoms

Anticipate that you may experience detox symptoms such as headaches, fatigue, irritability, digestive disturbances, or increased mucus production during the cleanse as your body releases accumulated toxins and metabolic waste. Mentally prepare yourself for these challenges and remind yourself that they are temporary and part of the cleansing process. Stay patient, compassionate, and gentle with yourself as you navigate the ups and downs of detoxification.

Conclusion

Preparing your body and mind for a 3-day herbal mucus cleanse involves careful planning, intention setting, education, dietary adjustments, hydration, stress management, and creating a supportive environment. By taking proactive steps to prepare for the cleanse, you can enhance its effectiveness, minimize potential detox symptoms, and maximize the benefits for respiratory health, immune function, and overall well-being. With dedication, mindfulness, and a spirit of self-care, you can embark on your herbal mucus cleanse journey with confidence and optimism.

CHAPTER SIX

Dr. Barbara's Approved Herbs and Herbal Remedies for the Cleanse

Dr. Barbara, a respected practitioner in herbal medicine and holistic healing, has carefully selected a range of herbs and herbal remedies to support the body's natural detoxification processes and promote respiratory health during the mucus cleanse. These herbs are chosen for their decongestant, expectorant, immune-supportive, and anti-inflammatory properties, as well as their ability to nourish and rejuvenate the body. In this guide, we'll explore Dr. Barbara's approved herbs and herbal remedies for the cleanse, along with their potential benefits and recommended usage.

1. Eucalyptus (Eucalyptus globulus)

Eucalyptus is a powerful decongestant and expectorant herb that helps to clear mucus from the respiratory tract and relieve congestion. It contains cineole, a compound with mucolytic properties that helps to break down mucus and facilitate its expulsion. Eucalyptus also has antimicrobial and anti-inflammatory properties, making it effective for relieving coughs, sinus congestion, and respiratory infections. Dr. Barbara may recommend inhaling eucalyptus essential oil, drinking eucalyptus tea, or using eucalyptus steam inhalation as part of the mucus cleanse.

2. Peppermint (Mentha piperita)

Peppermint is a cooling and soothing herb that can help to alleviate respiratory congestion, sinus pressure, and coughing. It contains menthol, a compound that acts as a natural decongestant and bronchodilator, helping to open up the airways and promote easier breathing. Peppermint also has antimicrobial and analgesic properties, making it useful for relieving sore throats and reducing inflammation in the respiratory tract. Dr. Barbara may recommend drinking peppermint tea, inhaling peppermint essential oil, or using peppermint steam inhalation to support respiratory health during the cleanse.

3. Ginger (Zingiber officinale)

Ginger is a warming and stimulating herb that has been used for centuries in traditional medicine to support respiratory health and digestion. It contains gingerol and other bioactive compounds that have antioxidant, anti-inflammatory, and immune-boosting properties. Ginger helps to thin mucus, reduce congestion, and alleviate coughing by promoting expectoration and clearing the respiratory passages. Dr. Barbara may recommend drinking ginger tea, chewing on fresh ginger root, or incorporating ginger into meals as part of the mucus cleanse.

4. Licorice Root (Glycyrrhiza glabra)

Licorice root is a demulcent herb that soothes and coats the mucous membranes of the respiratory tract, providing relief from irritation, inflammation, and coughing. It contains glycyrrhizin, a compound with expectorant and anti-inflammatory properties that help to loosen mucus and reduce congestion. Licorice root also has immune-modulating effects, making it useful for supporting immune function during the cleanse. Dr. Barbara may recommend drinking licorice root tea or taking licorice root supplements as part of the mucus cleanse.

5. Marshmallow Root (Althaea officinalis)

Marshmallow root is a mucilaginous herb that forms a soothing gel-like substance when mixed with water, which helps to coat and protect the mucous membranes of the respiratory tract. It contains polysaccharides and other compounds that have demulcent, anti-inflammatory, and expectorant properties, making it effective for relieving coughs, sore throats, and respiratory congestion. Marshmallow root also helps to hydrate and soften mucus, making it easier to expel from the body. Dr. Barbara may recommend drinking marshmallow root tea or taking marshmallow root supplements to support respiratory health during the cleanse.

6. Nettle Leaf (Urtica dioica)

Nettle leaf is a nutritive herb that is rich in vitamins, minerals, and antioxidants, making it an excellent addition to the mucus cleanse for supporting overall health and vitality. It has astringent and anti-inflammatory properties that help to reduce excess mucus production and alleviate respiratory congestion. Nettle leaf also supports immune function and helps to strengthen the body's defenses against infections. Dr. Barbara may recommend drinking nettle leaf tea or taking nettle leaf supplements as part of the mucus cleanse.

7. Mullein (Verbascum thapsus)

Mullein is a gentle yet effective herb that has been used traditionally to support respiratory health and relieve congestion. It contains saponins and mucilage, which have expectorant and demulcent properties that help to loosen mucus and soothe irritated respiratory tissues. Mullein also has antimicrobial and anti-inflammatory properties, making it useful for alleviating coughs, bronchitis, and respiratory infections. Dr. Barbara may recommend drinking mullein tea or using mullein leaf infusions as part of the mucus cleanse.

8. Garlic (Allium sativum)

Garlic is a potent antimicrobial and immune-modulating herb that can help to fight off infections and support respiratory health during the mucus cleanse. It contains allicin and other sulfur compounds that have antibacterial, antiviral, and antifungal properties, making it effective for combating respiratory infections and reducing inflammation in the respiratory tract.

Garlic also helps to stimulate immune function and enhance the body's natural defenses against pathogens. Dr. Barbara may recommend incorporating raw or cooked garlic into meals or taking garlic supplements to support respiratory health during the cleanse.

Conclusion

Dr. Barbara's approved herbs and herbal remedies for the mucus cleanse are carefully selected for their ability to support respiratory health, alleviate congestion, promote expectoration, and boost immune function. These herbs work synergistically to clear excess mucus from the body, relieve respiratory symptoms, and enhance overall well-being. By incorporating these herbs into your cleanse regimen under the guidance of a qualified healthcare provider or herbalist, you can optimize the detoxification process and experience the benefits of improved respiratory health and vitality.

CHAPTER SEVEN

Sample Meal Plans and Recipes for the 3-Day Cleanse

Embarking on a 3-day cleanse requires careful planning to ensure that your body receives nourishing, detoxifying foods that support the elimination of toxins and promote overall health and well-being. Incorporating a variety of fresh, whole foods and herbal remedies can enhance the effectiveness of the cleanse and help you feel energized and revitalized. Here are sample meal plans and recipes for each day of the cleanse:

Day 1:

Breakfast:

- Green Smoothie
    - Ingredients:
        - 1 cup spinach or kale
        - 1/2 banana
        - 1/2 cup frozen berries
        - 1 tablespoon chia seeds
        - 1 cup almond milk or coconut water

- Instructions: Blend all ingredients until smooth and creamy.

Lunch:

- Quinoa Salad with Roasted Vegetables

  - Ingredients:

    - 1 cup cooked quinoa

    - Assorted roasted vegetables (such as bell peppers, zucchini, and carrots)

    - Handful of fresh herbs (such as parsley or cilantro)

    - Lemon vinaigrette (made with olive oil, lemon juice, garlic, and Dijon mustard)

  - Instructions: Toss cooked quinoa and roasted vegetables with fresh herbs and lemon vinaigrette.

Dinner:

- Lentil Soup

  - Ingredients:

    - 1 cup dried lentils

    - Assorted vegetables (such as onions, carrots, celery, and garlic)

    - Vegetable broth

- Herbs and spices (such as cumin, turmeric, and thyme)

- Instructions: Cook lentils and vegetables in vegetable broth until tender. Season with herbs and spices to taste.

Day 2:

Breakfast:

- Overnight Oats

    - Ingredients:

        - 1/2 cup rolled oats

        - 1/2 cup almond milk

        - 1/2 cup Greek yogurt

        - 1 tablespoon chia seeds

        - Fresh berries and sliced bananas for topping

    - Instructions: Mix oats, almond milk, Greek yogurt, and chia seeds in a jar. Refrigerate overnight. Serve topped with fresh berries and sliced bananas.

Lunch:

- Mixed Greens Salad with Grilled Chicken

    - Ingredients:

- Mixed greens (such as spinach, arugula, and romaine)

  - Grilled chicken breast

  - Sliced cucumbers, cherry tomatoes, and bell peppers

  - Balsamic vinaigrette dressing

- Instructions: Toss mixed greens, grilled chicken, and vegetables with balsamic vinaigrette dressing.

Dinner:

- Stir-Fried Tofu with Vegetables

  - Ingredients:

    - Firm tofu, cubed

    - Assorted vegetables (such as broccoli, bell peppers, and snap peas)

    - Soy sauce or tamari

    - Garlic and ginger, minced

    - Sesame oil

  - Instructions: Stir-fry tofu and vegetables in sesame oil with garlic and ginger. Season with soy sauce or tamari.

Day 3:

Breakfast:

- Berry and Spinach Smoothie Bowl

    - Ingredients:

        - 1 cup spinach

        - 1/2 cup frozen berries

        - 1/2 banana

        - 1/4 cup Greek yogurt

        - Toppings: granola, sliced almonds, shredded coconut

    - Instructions: Blend spinach, berries, banana, and Greek yogurt until smooth. Pour into a bowl and top with granola, almonds, and coconut.

Lunch:

- Quinoa Stuffed Bell Peppers

    - Ingredients:

        - Bell peppers, halved and seeded

        - Cooked quinoa

        - Black beans

        - Corn

- Salsa

- Shredded cheese (optional)

- Instructions: Fill bell pepper halves with cooked quinoa, black beans, corn, and salsa. Top with shredded cheese if desired. Bake until peppers are tender.

Dinner:

- Vegetable and Chickpea Curry

  - Ingredients:

    - Assorted vegetables (such as onions, carrots, bell peppers, and cauliflower)

    - Cooked chickpeas

    - Curry paste or powder

    - Coconut milk

    - Fresh cilantro for garnish

  - Instructions: Sauté vegetables and chickpeas in curry paste or powder. Add coconut milk and simmer until vegetables are tender. Serve over rice and garnish with fresh cilantro.

Snacks:

- Fresh fruit (such as apples, oranges, or grapes)

- Raw vegetables with hummus

- Herbal teas (such as peppermint, ginger, or chamomile)

Hydration:

- Drink plenty of water throughout the day to stay hydrated and support the body's detoxification processes. You can also enjoy herbal teas or infused water with lemon, cucumber, and mint for added flavor and hydration.

By following these sample meal plans and recipes, you can nourish your body with nutrient-dense foods and herbal remedies that support the cleanse and promote overall health and well-being. Adjust portion sizes and ingredients based on your individual preferences and dietary needs, and consult with a healthcare provider or nutritionist if you have any specific concerns or medical conditions.

CHAPTER EIGHT

Incorporating herbal teas and supplements

Incorporating herbal teas and supplements can enhance the results of your cleanse by supporting detoxification, boosting immunity, and promoting overall health and well-being. Herbal teas provide hydration and deliver therapeutic compounds that support various aspects of the cleansing process, while supplements offer concentrated doses of key nutrients and herbal extracts to optimize detoxification pathways. Here's how to incorporate herbal teas and supplements for enhanced results during your cleanse:

1. Herbal Teas:

Peppermint Tea: Peppermint tea is soothing to the digestive system and helps alleviate bloating and gas, making it an excellent choice for supporting digestive health during the cleanse. Drink peppermint tea between meals to aid digestion and promote overall comfort.

Ginger Tea: Ginger tea has potent anti-inflammatory and digestive properties that help soothe the digestive tract, reduce nausea, and promote detoxification. Enjoy ginger tea before meals to stimulate digestion and support detoxification pathways.

Dandelion Root Tea: Dandelion root tea is a natural diuretic that helps flush toxins from the body by promoting urination. It also supports liver health and digestion, making it a valuable addition to your cleanse regimen. Drink dandelion root tea in the morning or evening to support detoxification and elimination.

Nettle Leaf Tea: Nettle leaf tea is rich in vitamins, minerals, and antioxidants that support overall health and vitality. It has diuretic properties that help flush toxins from the body and supports kidney function. Enjoy nettle leaf tea throughout the day as a nourishing and detoxifying beverage.

Licorice Root Tea: Licorice root tea has anti-inflammatory and soothing properties that help alleviate respiratory congestion, sore throat, and coughing. It also supports adrenal health and may help balance cortisol levels during times of stress. Drink licorice root tea as needed to support respiratory health and comfort.

2. Herbal Supplements:

Milk Thistle: Milk thistle is a powerful herb that supports liver health and detoxification. It contains silymarin, a compound with antioxidant and anti-inflammatory properties that help protect the liver from damage and promote the elimination of toxins. Take milk thistle supplements daily to support liver function during the cleanse.

N-Acetyl Cysteine (NAC): N-Acetyl Cysteine (NAC) is an amino acid that supports glutathione production, a key antioxidant that plays a crucial role in detoxification. NAC helps protect against oxidative stress and supports liver health by promoting the breakdown and elimination of toxins. Take NAC supplements daily to support detoxification pathways.

Probiotics: Probiotics are beneficial bacteria that support digestive health and immune function. They help maintain a healthy balance of gut flora, which is essential for proper digestion, nutrient absorption, and detoxification. Take a high-quality probiotic supplement daily to support gut health and overall well-being during the cleanse.

Vitamin C: Vitamin C is a powerful antioxidant that supports immune function and detoxification. It helps neutralize free radicals and supports the production of glutathione, an important antioxidant involved in liver detoxification. Take vitamin C supplements daily to support immune function and detoxification pathways.

Turmeric: Turmeric is a potent anti-inflammatory herb that supports liver health and detoxification. It contains curcumin, a compound with antioxidant and anti-inflammatory properties that help protect the liver from damage and promote the elimination of toxins. Take turmeric supplements daily to support liver function and reduce inflammation during the cleanse.

3. Timing and Dosage:

Follow the recommended dosage instructions for each herbal supplement and consult with a healthcare provider or herbalist if you have any questions or concerns. Take supplements with meals to enhance absorption and minimize the risk of digestive upset.

Incorporate herbal teas into your daily routine by enjoying them between meals or as a soothing beverage before bedtime. Experiment with different herbal teas to find combinations that support your individual needs and preferences.

4. Hydration and Supportive Practices:

Stay hydrated throughout the cleanse by drinking plenty of water, herbal teas, and other hydrating beverages. Hydration is essential for supporting detoxification and promoting overall health and well-being.

In addition to herbal teas and supplements, incorporate supportive practices such as meditation, deep breathing exercises, yoga, and gentle exercise to reduce stress, support relaxation, and enhance detoxification.

By incorporating herbal teas and supplements into your cleanse regimen, you can enhance detoxification, support immune function, and promote overall health and well-being. Experiment with different herbs and supplements to find combinations that work best for you, and consult with a healthcare provider or herbalist if you have any specific concerns or medical conditions.

CHAPTER NINE

Managing detox symptoms

Managing detox symptoms and supporting your body's natural processes are essential aspects of a successful cleanse. Detoxification can sometimes lead to temporary discomfort as the body eliminates toxins and adjusts to dietary changes. However, there are several strategies you can employ to minimize symptoms, support detoxification, and promote overall well-being during the cleanse:

1. Stay Hydrated:

- Drink plenty of water throughout the day to support hydration and flush toxins from the body.

- Herbal teas, such as peppermint, ginger, and dandelion root tea, can also support hydration and promote detoxification.

2. Eat Nutrient-Dense Foods:

- Consume a variety of whole foods, including fruits, vegetables, whole grains, legumes, nuts, and seeds, to provide essential nutrients that support detoxification and overall health.

- Incorporate foods rich in antioxidants, such as berries, leafy greens, and cruciferous vegetables, to help neutralize free radicals and reduce oxidative stress.

3. Support Liver Health:

- The liver plays a central role in detoxification. Support liver function by consuming foods and herbs that promote liver health, such as garlic, turmeric, beets, and leafy greens.

- Milk thistle supplements can also support liver health and aid in detoxification.

4. Practice Gentle Exercise:

- Engage in gentle exercise, such as walking, yoga, or tai chi, to support circulation, lymphatic drainage, and overall detoxification.

- Avoid strenuous exercise during the cleanse, as it may deplete energy reserves and exacerbate detox symptoms.

5. Practice Stress Reduction Techniques:

- Stress can impair detoxification pathways and exacerbate symptoms. Practice stress reduction techniques, such as meditation, deep breathing exercises, and progressive muscle relaxation, to promote relaxation and support detoxification.

6. Get Adequate Rest:

- Prioritize sleep and aim for 7-9 hours of quality sleep per night to support the body's natural healing processes and promote overall well-being.

- Allow yourself time for rest and relaxation during the cleanse to conserve energy and support detoxification.

7. Listen to Your Body:

- Pay attention to your body's signals and adjust your cleanse regimen as needed based on how you're feeling.

- If you experience severe or persistent symptoms, such as nausea, dizziness, or severe fatigue, consult with a healthcare provider to ensure your safety and well-being.

8. Support Digestive Health:

- Consume foods that support digestive health, such as probiotic-rich foods like yogurt, kefir, sauerkraut, and kombucha.

- Incorporate fiber-rich foods, such as fruits, vegetables, whole grains, and legumes, to support regular bowel movements and eliminate toxins from the body.

9. Consider Herbal Supplements:

- Certain herbal supplements, such as probiotics, digestive enzymes, and fiber supplements, can support digestive health and alleviate detox symptoms.

- Consult with a healthcare provider or herbalist to determine which supplements may be beneficial for you during the cleanse.

10. Gradually Reintroduce Foods:

- After completing the cleanse, gradually reintroduce foods into your diet to avoid overwhelming your digestive system and minimize the risk of digestive upset.

- Start with easily digestible foods, such as steamed vegetables, soups, and smoothies, before gradually reintroducing other foods.

By implementing these strategies, you can effectively manage detox symptoms, support your body's natural processes, and promote overall well-being during the cleanse. Remember to listen to your body, prioritize self-care, and consult with a healthcare provider if you have any concerns or medical conditions.

CHAPTER TEN

Maintaining a mucus-free lifestyle after the detox

Maintaining a mucus-free lifestyle after completing the cleanse requires long-term commitment to healthy habits and mindful choices that support respiratory health, immune function, and overall well-being. While the cleanse can provide a reset and jumpstart to healthier habits, it's essential to continue prioritizing self-care and making sustainable lifestyle changes to prevent the buildup of excess mucus and promote optimal health. Here are some long-term strategies for maintaining a mucus-free lifestyle after the cleanse:

1. Adopt a Balanced Diet:

- Focus on consuming a balanced diet rich in whole foods, including fruits, vegetables, whole grains, legumes, nuts, seeds, and lean proteins.

- Limit or avoid processed foods, refined sugars, artificial additives, and inflammatory substances that can contribute to mucus production and overall toxicity in the body.

2. Hydrate Adequately:

- Drink plenty of water throughout the day to stay hydrated and support the body's natural detoxification processes.

- Incorporate herbal teas, such as peppermint, ginger, and chamomile tea, which have decongestant and soothing properties, into your daily routine.

3. Manage Stress:

- Practice stress reduction techniques, such as meditation, deep breathing exercises, yoga, and mindfulness practices, to reduce stress levels and support overall well-being.

- Prioritize self-care activities that promote relaxation and rejuvenation, such as spending time in nature, engaging in hobbies, and connecting with loved ones.

4. Support Digestive Health:

- Maintain digestive health by consuming fiber-rich foods, probiotic-rich foods, and prebiotic-rich foods that support gut microbiome balance and regular bowel movements.

- Avoid overeating and practice mindful eating habits, such as chewing food thoroughly and eating slowly, to support digestion and nutrient absorption.

5. Incorporate Herbal Remedies:

- Continue incorporating herbal remedies and supplements that support respiratory health and immune function into your daily routine.

- Consider incorporating herbs such as turmeric, ginger, garlic, and echinacea into your diet or supplement regimen to support immune function and reduce inflammation.

6. Practice Regular Physical Activity:

- Engage in regular physical activity, such as walking, jogging, cycling, swimming, or yoga, to support circulation, lymphatic drainage, and overall detoxification.

- Find activities that you enjoy and incorporate them into your daily routine to promote physical fitness and overall well-being.

7. Prioritize Sleep:

- Aim for 7-9 hours of quality sleep per night to support the body's natural healing processes, immune function, and overall well-being.

- Establish a regular sleep schedule and create a relaxing bedtime routine to promote restful sleep and optimize sleep quality.

8. Minimize Exposure to Environmental Toxins:

- Minimize exposure to environmental toxins and pollutants, such as cigarette smoke, air pollution, household chemicals, and allergens, which can irritate the respiratory tract and contribute to mucus production.

- Use natural and eco-friendly cleaning products, air purifiers, and filters to reduce indoor air pollution and create a healthier living environment.

9. Practice Mindful Eating:

- Practice mindful eating by paying attention to hunger and fullness cues, savoring each bite, and cultivating gratitude for the nourishment provided by food.

- Be mindful of portion sizes and avoid overeating, which can strain the digestive system and contribute to mucus production.

10. Listen to Your Body:

- Listen to your body's signals and honor its needs by tuning into physical sensations, emotions, and intuition.

- Pay attention to how different foods, activities, and lifestyle choices affect your health and well-being, and make adjustments accordingly.

By incorporating these long-term strategies into your daily routine, you can maintain a mucus-free lifestyle and support respiratory health, immune function, and overall well-being over the long term. Remember that small, sustainable changes add up over time and lead to lasting improvements in health and vitality.

BONUS: SOME ESSENTIAL HERBAL REMEDIES TO KNOW

Bromide Plus Powder:

Definition: Bromide Plus Powder is a dietary supplement formulated to support thyroid health and promote overall well-being. It typically contains a blend of herbs and minerals that are believed to have beneficial effects on thyroid function.

Ingredients: Bromide Plus Powder often contains a combination of herbs such as bladderwrack, sea moss, and burdock root, along with minerals like iodine and potassium phosphate. These ingredients are thought to support thyroid function and maintain optimal iodine levels in the body.

How to Prepare: Bromide Plus Powder is usually mixed with water or juice to create a drinkable solution. It's important to follow the instructions on the product label for dosage and preparation.

Dosage: The dosage of Bromide Plus Powder can vary depending on the specific product and individual needs. It's crucial to consult with a healthcare professional or follow the recommended dosage on the product label to avoid potential side effects.

How to Use: Bromide Plus Powder is typically taken orally by mixing the recommended dosage with water or juice. It's important to shake or stir the mixture well before consuming it to ensure even distribution of the ingredients.

Side Effects: While Bromide Plus Powder is generally considered safe when used as directed, some individuals may experience side effects such as digestive discomfort or allergic reactions to certain ingredients. It's essential to consult with a healthcare provider before starting any new supplement regimen, especially if you have underlying health conditions or are taking medications.

Bugleweed:

Definition: Bugleweed, also known as Lycopusvirginicus, is a perennial herb native to North America and Europe. It has been used in traditional medicine to treat various conditions, including hyperthyroidism, anxiety, and insomnia.

Ingredients: Bugleweed contains several active compounds, including lithospermic acid, phenolic acids, and flavonoids. These compounds are believed to contribute to the herb's medicinal properties, particularly its ability to regulate thyroid function.

How to Prepare: Bugleweed is commonly consumed as a tea or tincture. To make tea, dried bugleweed leaves and flowers are steeped in hot water for several minutes before being strained and consumed. Tinctures are prepared by steeping the herb in alcohol or vinegar to extract its active compounds.

Dosage: The appropriate dosage of bugleweed can vary depending on factors such as age, health status, and the specific preparation being used. It's important to follow the recommended dosage on the product label or consult with a qualified herbalist or healthcare professional for personalized guidance.

How to Use: Bugleweed tea or tincture is typically taken orally. It can be consumed on its own or mixed with honey or other herbal teas for added flavor.

Side Effects: While bugleweed is generally considered safe for most people when used in moderation, excessive intake may cause digestive upset or allergic reactions in some individuals. Pregnant or breastfeeding women should avoid bugleweed due to its potential to stimulate uterine contractions. As with any herbal remedy, it's important to consult with a healthcare provider before using bugleweed, especially if you have underlying health conditions or are taking medications.

Burdock:

Definition: Burdock, scientifically known as Arctium lappa, is a biennial plant native to Europe and Asia but now found worldwide. It's part of the Asteraceae family and has been used for centuries in traditional medicine and culinary practices.

Ingredients: Burdock contains various nutrients, including carbohydrates, fiber, vitamins (such as vitamin B6, folate, and vitamin C), and minerals (including potassium, magnesium, and manganese). It also contains active compounds such as polyphenols and volatile oils.

How to Prepare: Burdock can be prepared and consumed in various ways. The roots, leaves, and seeds are all utilized for different purposes. The root is commonly used in cooking, herbal teas, tinctures, and supplements, while the leaves and seeds are sometimes used in herbal preparations.

Dosage: The appropriate dosage of burdock root can vary depending on the specific form and intended use. For culinary purposes, there are no strict dosage guidelines, but for supplements or herbal remedies, it's essential to follow the recommended dosage on the product label or consult with a healthcare professional.

How to Use: Burdock root can be used in cooking by peeling, slicing, and adding it to soups, stews, stir-fries, or salads. It can also be brewed into a tea or used to make tinctures or extracts for medicinal purposes. Some people may also take burdock root supplements in capsule or powder form.

Side Effects: While burdock is generally considered safe for most people when consumed in moderate amounts, some individuals may experience allergic reactions or digestive upset. Additionally, burdock may interact with certain medications or have adverse effects in individuals with certain health conditions, such as diabetes or allergies to plants in the Asteraceae family. It's important to consult with a healthcare provider before using burdock, especially if you have underlying health conditions or are taking medications.

Cascara Sagrada:

Definition: Cascara Sagrada, scientifically known as Rhamnus purshiana, is a species of buckthorn native to western North America. It has been used traditionally as a laxative and to promote bowel regularity.

Ingredients: The primary active ingredients in cascara sagrada are anthraquinone glycosides, particularly cascarosides A and B. These compounds stimulate peristalsis in the colon, leading to increased bowel movements.

How to Prepare: Cascara sagrada is typically prepared as an herbal tea, tincture, or capsule. To make tea, dried cascara sagrada bark is steeped in hot water for several minutes before being strained and consumed. Tinctures are prepared by steeping the bark in alcohol to extract its active compounds.

Dosage: The appropriate dosage of cascara sagrada can vary depending on the specific preparation and intended use. It's important to follow the recommended dosage on the product label or consult with a healthcare professional for personalized guidance.

How to Use: Cascara sagrada tea or tincture is typically taken orally. It's important to start with a low dose and gradually increase if needed to avoid potential side effects such as cramping or diarrhea.

Side Effects: Cascara sagrada is considered safe for short-term use when used as directed. However, long-term or excessive use may lead to dependence, electrolyte imbalance, or dehydration. It may also interact with certain medications or have adverse effects in individuals with certain health conditions. It's important to use cascara sagrada under the guidance of a healthcare professional and to discontinue use if any adverse effects occur.

Cell Food:

Definition: Cell Food is a dietary supplement marketed as a highly oxygenating and alkalizing formula. It's claimed to support overall health and vitality by providing essential nutrients and oxygen to the cells.

Ingredients: The exact ingredients of Cell Food can vary depending on the brand, but it typically contains a proprietary blend of minerals, enzymes, electrolytes, and trace elements. Some common ingredients may include purified water, dissolved oxygen, seawater extract, and plant-based enzymes.

How to Prepare: Cell Food is usually available in liquid form and is typically taken orally. It can be consumed directly or diluted in water or juice before consumption.

Dosage: The dosage of Cell Food can vary depending on the specific product and individual needs. It's important to follow the recommended dosage on the product label or consult with a healthcare professional for personalized guidance.

How to Use: Cell Food is typically taken orally, either directly or mixed into water or juice. It's important to shake the bottle well before use and to store it according to the manufacturer's instructions.

Side Effects: Cell Food is generally considered safe for most people when used as directed. However, some individuals may experience mild digestive upset or allergic reactions to certain ingredients. It's essential to consult with a healthcare provider before starting any new supplement regimen, especially if you have underlying health conditions or are taking medications.

Chaparral:

Definition: Chaparral, scientifically known as Larrea tridentata, is a shrub native to the southwestern United States and northern Mexico. It has been used for centuries by Native American tribes for its medicinal properties and is commonly used in herbal medicine today.

Ingredients: Chaparral contains several bioactive compounds, including nordihydroguaiaretic acid (NDGA), flavonoids, lignans, and volatile oils. NDGA is believed to be the primary active compound responsible for many of chaparral's therapeutic effects.

How to Prepare: Chaparral can be prepared and consumed in various forms, including teas, tinctures, capsules, and topical preparations. To make tea, dried chaparral leaves are steeped in hot water for several minutes before being strained and consumed. Tinctures are prepared by steeping the herb in alcohol or vinegar to extract its active compounds.

Dosage: The appropriate dosage of chaparral can vary depending on the specific form and intended use. It's important to follow the recommended dosage on the product label or consult with a healthcare professional for personalized guidance.

How to Use: Chaparral tea or tincture is typically taken orally. It can also be applied topically to the skin for certain conditions. It's important to use chaparral products as directed and to discontinue use if any adverse effects occur.

Side Effects: Chaparral is generally considered safe for most people when used in moderate amounts. However, excessive intake or prolonged use may lead to liver toxicity or other adverse effects. It may also interact with certain medications or have adverse effects in individuals with certain health conditions. It's important to use chaparral under the guidance of a healthcare professional and to discontinue use if any adverse effects occur.

Cocolmeca:

Definition: Cocolmeca, also known as Smilax ornata or sarsaparilla, is a flowering vine native to Mexico and Central America. It has been used traditionally in Mexican and Central American folk medicine for its purported medicinal properties.

Ingredients: Cocolmeca contains various bioactive compounds, including saponins, flavonoids, and plant sterols. These compounds are believed to contribute to the herb's medicinal properties, including its potential as a diuretic, blood purifier, and anti-inflammatory agent.

How to Prepare: Cocolmeca is commonly prepared and consumed as an herbal tea or decoction. To make tea, dried cocolmeca roots or leaves are steeped in hot water for several minutes before being strained and consumed. Decoctions involve boiling the roots or leaves in water to extract their active compounds.

Dosage: The appropriate dosage of cocolmeca can vary depending on factors such as age, health status, and the specific preparation being used. It's important to follow the recommended dosage on the product label or consult with a qualified herbalist or healthcare professional for personalized guidance.

How to Use: Cocolmeca tea or decoction is typically taken orally. It can also be used topically for certain skin conditions. It's important to use cocolmeca products as directed and to discontinue use if any adverse effects occur.

Side Effects: Cocolmeca is generally considered safe for most people when used in moderate amounts. However, excessive intake may lead to digestive upset or other adverse effects. It may also interact with certain medications or have adverse effects in individuals with certain health conditions. It's important to use cocolmeca under the guidance of a healthcare professional and to discontinue use if any adverse effects occur.

Contribo:

Definition: Contribo, also known as Aristolochiatrilobata, is a vine native to the Caribbean and Central America. It has been used traditionally in folk medicine for various purposes, including as a remedy for digestive issues, inflammation, and pain relief.

Ingredients: Contribo contains several bioactive compounds, including aristolochic acids, flavonoids, and alkaloids. These compounds are believed to contribute to the herb's medicinal properties, including its potential as an anti-inflammatory and analgesic agent.

How to Prepare: Contribo is typically prepared and consumed as an herbal tea or decoction. To make tea, dried contribo leaves or stems are steeped in hot water for several minutes before being strained and consumed. Decoctions involve boiling the leaves or stems in water to extract their active compounds.

Dosage: The appropriate dosage of contribo can vary depending on factors such as age, health status, and the specific preparation being used. It's important to follow the recommended dosage on the product label or consult with a qualified herbalist or healthcare professional for personalized guidance.

How to Use: Contribo tea or decoction is typically taken orally. It's important to use contribo products as directed and to discontinue use if any adverse effects occur.

Side Effects: Contribo contains aristolochic acids, which have been associated with serious adverse effects, including kidney damage and cancer. Due to these safety concerns, the use of contribo is highly discouraged, and it's important to avoid products containing aristolochic acids. Individuals should seek alternative remedies for their health needs.

Dandelion Root:

Definition: Dandelion, scientifically known as Taraxacum officinale, is a common flowering plant found worldwide. While often considered a pesky weed, dandelion has a long history of use in traditional medicine for its various health benefits.

Ingredients: Dandelion root contains several bioactive compounds, including sesquiterpene lactones, triterpenes, flavonoids, and polysaccharides. These compounds are believed to contribute to the herb's medicinal properties, including its potential as a diuretic, digestive aid, and liver tonic.

How to Prepare: Dandelion root can be prepared and consumed in various forms, including teas, tinctures, capsules, and extracts. To make tea, dried dandelion root is steeped in hot water for several minutes before being strained and consumed. Tinctures are prepared by steeping the root in alcohol or vinegar to extract its active compounds.

Dosage: The appropriate dosage of dandelion root can vary depending on factors such as age, health status, and the specific preparation being used. It's important to follow the recommended dosage on the product label or consult with a qualified herbalist or healthcare professional for personalized guidance.

How to Use: Dandelion root tea, tincture, or capsules are typically taken orally. It's important to use dandelion root products as directed and to discontinue use if any adverse effects occur.

Side Effects: Dandelion root is generally considered safe for most people when used in moderate amounts. However, some individuals may experience allergic reactions or digestive upset. It may also interact with certain medications or have adverse effects in individuals with certain health conditions. It's important to use dandelion root under the guidance of a healthcare professional and to discontinue use if any adverse effects occur.

Green Food Plus:

Definition: Green Food Plus is a dietary supplement formulated to provide a concentrated source of nutrients derived from various green plants. It's designed to support overall health and well-being by delivering essential vitamins, minerals, antioxidants, and phytonutrients.

Ingredients: Green Food Plus typically contains a blend of powdered green vegetables, grasses, algae, and other plant-based ingredients. Common ingredients may include wheatgrass, barley grass, spirulina, chlorella, alfalfa, kale, spinach, and broccoli, among others.

How to Prepare: Green Food Plus is usually available in powder form and can be mixed with water, juice, or smoothies. It's important to follow the recommended dosage on the product label and to consume it as part of a balanced diet.

Dosage: The appropriate dosage of Green Food Plus can vary depending on the specific product and individual needs. It's important to follow the recommended dosage on the product label or consult with a healthcare professional for personalized guidance.

How to Use: Green Food Plus powder is typically mixed with water, juice, or smoothies and consumed orally. It's often taken once or twice daily, preferably with meals, to maximize nutrient absorption.

Side Effects: Green Food Plus is generally considered safe for most people when used as directed. However, some individuals may experience digestive upset or allergic reactions to certain ingredients. It's important to consult with a healthcare provider before starting any new supplement regimen, especially if you have underlying health conditions or are taking medications.

Guaco:

Definition: Guaco, also known as Mikania cordata or Mikania glomerata, is a medicinal plant native to Central and South America. It has a long history of use in traditional medicine for its potential therapeutic properties.

Ingredients: Guaco contains several bioactive compounds, including coumarins, flavonoids, tannins, and saponins. These compounds are believed to contribute to the herb's medicinal properties, including its potential as an expectorant, anti-inflammatory, and antispasmodic agent.

How to Prepare: Guaco is typically prepared and consumed as an herbal tea or infusion. To make tea, dried guaco leaves are steeped in hot water for several minutes before being strained and consumed.

Dosage: The appropriate dosage of guaco can vary depending on factors such as age, health status, and the specific preparation being used. It's important to follow the recommended dosage on the product label or consult with a qualified herbalist or healthcare professional for personalized guidance.

How to Use: Guaco tea is typically taken orally. It can be consumed on its own or mixed with honey or other herbal teas for added flavor.

Side Effects: Guaco is generally considered safe for most people when used in moderate amounts. However, some individuals may experience allergic reactions or digestive upset. It may also interact with certain medications or have adverse effects in individuals with certain health conditions. It's important to use guaco under the guidance of a healthcare professional and to discontinue use if any adverse effects occur.

Herban Iron:

Definition: Herban Iron is a dietary supplement designed to provide an easily absorbable form of iron to support healthy iron levels in the body. It's particularly beneficial for individuals with iron deficiency or anemia.

Ingredients: Herban Iron typically contains iron in the form of ferrous bisglycinate, which is a highly bioavailable and gentle form of iron that is less likely to cause digestive upset or constipation compared to other forms of iron. It may also contain other ingredients such as vitamin C to enhance iron absorption.

How to Prepare: Herban Iron is usually available in capsule or liquid form. Capsules are taken orally with water, while liquid forms may be mixed with water or juice before consumption. It's important to follow the recommended dosage on the product label.

Dosage: The appropriate dosage of Herban Iron depends on factors such as age, gender, and the severity of iron deficiency. It's important to consult with a healthcare professional to determine the correct dosage for individual needs.

How to Use: Herban Iron capsules are typically taken orally with water, while liquid forms may be mixed with water or juice before consumption. It's important to take Herban Iron as directed and to avoid taking it with dairy products, antacids, or other substances that may interfere with iron absorption.

Side Effects: While Herban Iron is generally considered safe for most people when used as directed, some individuals may experience mild side effects such as gastrointestinal discomfort or constipation. It's important to consult with a healthcare professional before starting any new supplement regimen, especially if you have underlying health conditions or are taking medications.

Hydrangea:

Definition: Hydrangea, scientifically known as Hydrangea arborescens, is a flowering shrub native to North America. It has been used traditionally in herbal medicine for its potential diuretic and anti-inflammatory properties.

Ingredients: Hydrangea contains several bioactive compounds, including saponins, flavonoids, and glycosides. These compounds are believed to contribute to the herb's medicinal properties, including its potential as a diuretic, kidney tonic, and anti-inflammatory agent.

How to Prepare: Hydrangea root is typically prepared and consumed as an herbal tea or tincture. To make tea, dried hydrangea root is steeped in hot water for several minutes before being strained and consumed. Tinctures are prepared by steeping the root in alcohol or vinegar to extract its active compounds.

Dosage: The appropriate dosage of hydrangea can vary depending on factors such as age, health status, and the specific preparation being used. It's important to follow the recommended dosage on the product label or consult with a qualified herbalist or healthcare professional for personalized guidance.

How to Use: Hydrangea tea or tincture is typically taken orally. It's important to use hydrangea products as directed and to discontinue use if any adverse effects occur.

Side Effects: Hydrangea is generally considered safe for most people when used in moderate amounts. However, some individuals may experience digestive upset or allergic reactions. It may also interact with certain medications or have adverse effects in individuals with certain health conditions. It's important to use hydrangea under the guidance of a healthcare professional and to discontinue use if any adverse effects occur.

Irish Moss:

Definition: Irish Moss, scientifically known as Chondrus crispus, is a species of red algae or seaweed native to the Atlantic coastlines of Europe and North America. It has been used for centuries in traditional Irish and Scottish cuisine, as well as in herbal medicine.

Ingredients: Irish Moss is rich in various nutrients, including iodine, sulfur compounds, vitamins (such as vitamin A, vitamin K, and vitamin B12), minerals (including calcium, magnesium, potassium, and sodium), and polysaccharides (such as carrageenan). These nutrients are believed to contribute to the herb's potential health benefits.

How to Prepare: Irish Moss is typically prepared by soaking it in water to rehydrate and soften it before use. It can be added to soups, stews, smoothies, desserts, and other dishes as a thickening agent or nutritional supplement.

Dosage: The appropriate dosage of Irish Moss can vary depending on factors such as age, health status, and the specific preparation being used. It's important to follow recipes or guidelines for culinary use and to consult with a healthcare professional for guidance on using Irish Moss as a dietary supplement.

How to Use: Irish Moss can be used in culinary applications to add thickness and nutritional value to dishes. It can also be consumed as a dietary supplement in the form of capsules, powders, or extracts.

Side Effects: Irish Moss is generally considered safe for most people when consumed in moderate amounts as part of a balanced diet. However, some individuals may be allergic to seaweed or carrageenan, a compound found in Irish Moss that is used as a food additive. It's important to discontinue use if any adverse effects occur and to consult with a healthcare professional if you have any concerns.

Red Clover:

Definition: Red clover, scientifically known as Trifolium pratense, is a flowering plant belonging to the legume family. It's native to Europe, Western Asia, and Northwest Africa but has been naturalized in many other regions. Red clover has been used in traditional medicine for various purposes, including its potential to support women's health and menopausal symptoms.

Ingredients: Red clover contains several bioactive compounds, including isoflavones (such as genistein and daidzein), flavonoids, and phytoestrogens. These compounds are believed to contribute to the herb's medicinal properties, including its potential as a hormone-balancing agent and its ability to support cardiovascular health.

How to Prepare: Red clover is typically prepared and consumed as an herbal tea or tincture. To make tea, dried red clover flowers are steeped in hot water for several minutes before being strained and consumed. Tinctures are prepared by steeping the flowers in alcohol or vinegar to extract their active compounds.

Dosage: The appropriate dosage of red clover can vary depending on factors such as age, health status, and the specific preparation being used. It's important to follow the recommended dosage on the product label or consult with a qualified herbalist or healthcare professional for personalized guidance.

How to Use: Red clover tea or tincture is typically taken orally. It's important to use red clover products as directed and to discontinue use if any adverse effects occur.

Side Effects: Red clover is generally considered safe for most people when used in moderate amounts. However, some individuals may experience allergic reactions or digestive upset. It may also interact with certain medications or have adverse effects in individuals with certain health conditions. It's important to use red clover under the guidance of a healthcare professional and to discontinue use if any adverse effects occur.

Red Raspberry:

Definition: Red raspberry, scientifically known as Rubus idaeus, is a species of raspberry native to Europe and northern Asia. It's widely cultivated for its delicious berries and has been used in traditional medicine for various purposes, including its potential to support women's health during pregnancy and childbirth.

Ingredients: Red raspberry contains several bioactive compounds, including flavonoids, ellagic acid, anthocyanins, and vitamin C. These compounds are believed to contribute to the herb's medicinal properties, including its potential as an antioxidant, anti-inflammatory, and uterine tonic.

How to Prepare: Red raspberry leaf is typically prepared and consumed as an herbal tea or infusion. To make tea, dried red raspberry leaves are steeped in hot water for several minutes before being strained and consumed.

Dosage: The appropriate dosage of red raspberry leaf can vary depending on factors such as age, health status, and the specific preparation being used. It's important to follow the recommended dosage on the product label or consult with a qualified herbalist or healthcare professional for personalized guidance.

How to Use: Red raspberry leaf tea is typically taken orally. It's often recommended for pregnant individuals in the later stages of pregnancy to support uterine health and prepare for childbirth. It's important to use red raspberry leaf products as directed and to discontinue use if any adverse effects occur.

Side Effects: Red raspberry leaf is generally considered safe for most people when used in moderate amounts. However, some individuals may experience allergic reactions or digestive upset. Pregnant individuals should consult with a healthcare professional before using red raspberry leaf, especially if they have any underlying health conditions or are taking medications. It's important to use red raspberry leaf under the guidance of a healthcare professional and to discontinue use if any adverse effects occur.

Tila:

Definition: Tila, also known as linden flower or lime blossom, refers to the flowers of the Tilia genus, primarily Tilia europaea and Tilia cordata. These trees are native to Europe, but they are also cultivated in other regions for their fragrant and medicinal flowers.

Ingredients: Tila flowers contain various bioactive compounds, including flavonoids, phenolic acids, and volatile oils. These compounds are believed to contribute to the herb's medicinal properties, including its potential as a mild sedative, anxiolytic, and anti-inflammatory agent.

How to Prepare: Tila flowers are typically prepared and consumed as an herbal tea or infusion. To make tea, dried tila flowers are steeped in hot water for several minutes before being strained and consumed.

Dosage: The appropriate dosage of tila can vary depending on factors such as age, health status, and the specific preparation being used. It's important to follow the recommended dosage on the product label or consult with a qualified herbalist or healthcare professional for personalized guidance.

How to Use: Tila tea is typically taken orally. It's often consumed in the evening as a calming bedtime beverage or during times of stress or anxiety. It's important to use tila products as directed and to discontinue use if any adverse effects occur.

Side Effects: Tila is generally considered safe for most people when used in moderate amounts. However, some individuals may experience allergic reactions or digestive upset. It may also interact with certain medications or have adverse effects in individuals with certain health conditions. It's important to use tila under the guidance of a healthcare professional and to discontinue use if any adverse effects occur.

Valerian:

Definition: Valerian, scientifically known as Valeriana officinalis, is a perennial flowering plant native to Europe and Asia. It has been used for centuries in traditional medicine for its potential calming and sedative effects.

Ingredients: Valerian root contains several bioactive compounds, including valerenic acid, valepotriates, and volatile oils. These compounds are believed to contribute to the herb's medicinal properties, including its potential as a sedative, anxiolytic, and sleep aid.

How to Prepare: Valerian root is typically prepared and consumed as an herbal tea, tincture, or capsule. To make tea, dried valerian root is steeped in hot water for several minutes before being strained and consumed. Tinctures are prepared by steeping the root in alcohol or vinegar to extract its active compounds.

Dosage: The appropriate dosage of valerian can vary depending on factors such as age, health status, and the specific preparation being used. It's important to follow the recommended dosage on the product label or consult with a qualified herbalist or healthcare professional for personalized guidance.

How to Use: Valerian tea, tincture, or capsules are typically taken orally. It's often consumed in the evening as a sleep aid or during times of stress or anxiety. It's important to use valerian products as directed and to discontinue use if any adverse effects occur.

Side Effects: Valerian is generally considered safe for most people when used in moderate amounts. However, some individuals may experience mild side effects such as drowsiness, headache, or gastrointestinal upset. It may also interact with certain medications or have adverse effects in individuals with certain health conditions. It's important to use valerian under the guidance of a healthcare professional and to discontinue use if any adverse effects occur.

Rhubarb:

Definition: Rhubarb, scientifically known as Rheum rhabarbarum, is a perennial plant cultivated for its edible stalks. While primarily used in culinary applications, rhubarb has also been utilized in traditional medicine for its potential health benefits, particularly for digestive health.

Ingredients: Rhubarb stalks contain various bioactive compounds, including anthraquinones (such as emodin and rhein), fiber, vitamins (such as vitamin K), and minerals (including calcium and potassium). These compounds are believed to contribute to the herb's medicinal properties, including its potential as a laxative and digestive aid.

How to Prepare: Rhubarb stalks are typically cooked before consumption, as the raw stalks are very tart and can be unpleasant to eat. They are often used in pies, crisps, jams, sauces, and other desserts, as well as in savory dishes. Rhubarb can also be used to make compotes, jams, and preserves.

Dosage: There is no specific dosage for rhubarb in culinary applications, as it is used as a food rather than a medicinal herb. However, when used for its potential laxative effects, it's important to consume rhubarb in moderation to avoid gastrointestinal upset.

How to Use: Rhubarb stalks can be chopped and cooked in various dishes, including pies, sauces, and jams. It's important to remove and discard the leaves, as they contain toxic compounds. When using rhubarb for its potential laxative effects, it's typically consumed as part of a cooked dish or in the form of a rhubarb-based herbal remedy.

Side Effects: Rhubarb stalks are generally safe for most people when consumed in moderate amounts as part of a balanced diet. However, excessive intake may lead to digestive upset or adverse effects due to the presence of oxalic acid, which can bind to calcium and form kidney stones in susceptible individuals. It's important to use rhubarb in moderation and to consult with a healthcare professional if you have any concerns or underlying health conditions.

Sarsaparilla:

Definition: Sarsaparilla refers to several species of plants belonging to the Smilax genus, including Smilax regelii and Smilax officinalis. It has been used historically in traditional medicine for its potential health benefits, particularly for its purported detoxifying and anti-inflammatory properties.

Ingredients: Sarsaparilla contains various bioactive compounds, including saponins (such as sarsaponin and smilagenin), flavonoids, phenolic acids, and sterols. These compounds are believed to contribute to the herb's medicinal properties, including its potential as a diuretic, blood purifier, and anti-inflammatory agent.

How to Prepare: Sarsaparilla root is typically prepared and consumed as an herbal tea, decoction, or tincture. To make tea, dried sarsaparilla root is steeped in hot water for several minutes before being strained and consumed. Decoctions involve boiling the root in water to extract its active compounds, while tinctures are prepared by steeping the root in alcohol or vinegar.

Dosage: The appropriate dosage of sarsaparilla can vary depending on factors such as age, health status, and the specific preparation being used. It's important to follow the recommended dosage on the product label or consult with a qualified herbalist or healthcare professional for personalized guidance.

How to Use: Sarsaparilla tea or tincture is typically taken orally. It's important to use sarsaparilla products as directed and to discontinue use if any adverse effects occur.

Side Effects: Sarsaparilla is generally considered safe for most people when used in moderate amounts. However, some individuals may experience allergic reactions or digestive upset. It may also interact with certain medications or have adverse effects in individuals with certain health conditions. It's important to use sarsaparilla under the guidance of a healthcare professional and to discontinue use if any adverse effects occur.

Irish Sea Moss:

Definition: Irish Sea Moss is a term often used interchangeably with Irish Moss, referring to the same species of red algae, Chondrus crispus. It's harvested from the rocky shores of the Atlantic coastlines of Europe and North America.

Ingredients: Irish Sea Moss shares the same nutritional profile as Irish Moss, containing iodine, vitamins, minerals, and polysaccharides. It's valued for its potential health benefits, including supporting thyroid function, boosting immune health, and promoting digestion.

How to Prepare: Irish Sea Moss is prepared in the same way as Irish Moss, by soaking it in water to rehydrate and soften it before use. It can be used in culinary applications or consumed as a dietary supplement.

Dosage: The dosage of Irish Sea Moss depends on the form and intended use. As a dietary supplement, it's important to follow the recommended dosage on the product label or consult with a healthcare professional for personalized guidance.

How to Use: Irish Sea Moss can be used in various culinary applications, including soups, smoothies, desserts, and sauces. It can also be consumed as a dietary supplement in the form of capsules, powders, or extracts.

Side Effects: Similar to Irish Moss, Irish Sea Moss is generally considered safe for most people when consumed in moderate amounts. However, individuals with seaweed allergies or sensitivities to carrageenan should exercise caution. It's important to discontinue use if any adverse effects occur and to consult with a healthcare professional if you have any concerns.

Lymphalin:

Definition: Lymphalin is a herbal supplement formulated to support lymphatic system health. The lymphatic system plays a crucial role in immune function and waste removal in the body, and Lymphalin is designed to promote its proper function.

Ingredients: Lymphalin typically contains a blend of herbs and botanical extracts known for their traditional use in supporting lymphatic system health. Common ingredients may include cleavers, red clover, echinacea, burdock root, and calendula, among others.

How to Prepare: Lymphalin is usually available in capsule or liquid form. Capsules are taken orally with water, while liquid forms may be mixed with water or juice before consumption. It's important to follow the recommended dosage on the product label.

Dosage: The appropriate dosage of Lymphalin can vary depending on the specific product and individual needs. It's important to follow the recommended dosage on the product label or consult with a healthcare professional for personalized guidance.

How to Use: Lymphalin capsules are typically taken orally with water, while liquid forms may be mixed with water or juice before consumption. It's often recommended to take Lymphalin on an empty stomach for optimal absorption.

Side Effects: Lymphalin is generally considered safe for most people when used as directed. However, some individuals may experience mild side effects such as gastrointestinal discomfort or allergic reactions to certain ingredients. It's important to consult with a healthcare provider before starting any new supplement regimen, especially if you have underlying health conditions or are taking medications.

Manjakani:

Definition: Manjakani, also known as Quercus infectoria or oak gall, is a natural substance derived from the oak tree. It has been used for centuries in traditional medicine for its potential health benefits, particularly for women's health and vaginal tightening.

Ingredients: Manjakani contains various bioactive compounds, including tannins, flavonoids, and gallic acid. These compounds are believed to contribute to the herb's medicinal properties, including its potential as an astringent and antiseptic agent.

How to Prepare: Manjakani is typically available in powder, capsule, or liquid extract form. It can be taken orally or used topically depending on the intended use. For vaginal tightening, manjakani may be applied topically as a gel or inserted into the vagina in capsule form.

Dosage: The appropriate dosage of manjakani can vary depending on factors such as age, health status, and the specific preparation being used. It's important to follow the recommended dosage on the product label or consult with a qualified herbalist or healthcare professional for personalized guidance.

How to Use: Manjakani can be taken orally or used topically depending on the intended use. It's important to use manjakani products as directed and to discontinue use if any adverse effects occur.

Side Effects: Manjakani is generally considered safe for most people when used in moderate amounts. However, some individuals may experience allergic reactions or skin irritation when used topically. It's important to use manjakani under the guidance of a healthcare professional and to discontinue use if any adverse effects occur.

THE END